Kettlebell Workouts

For

Beginners

David Lynch

Copyright © 2014 David Lynch

All rights reserved.

No part of this book may be reproduced in any form or by any electronic or mechanical means, including information storage and retrieval systems, without prior permission of the publisher and author.

ISBN: 1495271498
ISBN-13: 978-1495271496

DEDICATION

Dedicated to you the reader - and the fitness you want to achieve. Never give up.

CONTENTS

Disclaimer & Precautions	i
Foreword	Pg 1
The History & Background of Kettlebells	Pg 2
Benefits of Kettlebells	Pg 4
Strength, flexibility and cardio all in one	
Suggested Kettlebell Weights	Pg 9
Other Equipment	Pg 12
Beginner's Kettlebell Workout Program	Pg 15
Two Handed Kettlebell Swing	
KB Swing Expert Tip #1	
KB Swing Expert Tip #2	
Kettlebell Deadlift	
Goblet Squat/Front Squat	
Kettlebell Woodman's Chop	
One Handed Kettlebell Swing	
Kettlebell Rotating Lunge	
Kettlebell Push-Up with Row	
Taking Your Training Further	Pg 43
Adding A Second Kettlebell	

Two-Arm Kettlebell Row

Alternating Kettlebell Press

Nutrition   Pg 50

   Universal Truth #1

   Universal Truth #2

   Universal Truth #3

   How Eating Fat Will Help You Get Fit

   Saturated Fats

   Monounsaturated Fats

   Polyunsaturated Fats

   Trans Fats

Conclusion   Pg 56

DISCLAIMER & PRECAUTIONS

Warning: Follow all directions printed and/or illustrated. Use caution and proper judgment at all times.

Always consult your physician prior to beginning any diet, exercise or physical training program. Should you experience serious pain, strain, or dizziness, stop immediately and seek the advice of a licensed health care professional.

Individuals involved in the production of this product, the author, publisher and distributor assume no responsibility for any injury or damage resulting from the execution or practice of the techniques presented.

Always keep safety in mind while practicing any of the techniques presented in this manual. This may include proper shoes, belts, gloves, and so on.

If you are unsure of how your body will react to certain exercise or foods/supplements, consult your physician before continuing.

FOREWORD

Firstly, well done on making a great decision!

Many people think about getting in shape or beginning their journey into a fitter, more agile, more alert version of themselves. Sadly, only a small percentage of those people ever do anything about realizing their goals. Just by taking the time to read this book, you have already begun to set yourself apart from the masses.

If at this point you feel hesitant or nervous about creating a new fitness routine for yourself, don't worry. Kettlebells are a fun and relatively simple tool that will help your body get to a high level of fitness very quickly. If you feel very apprehensive, console yourself that many people are able to lose weight and tone up with just one of the kettlebell exercises shown here. There has been some controversy around that move, which makes for an interesting read—but one thing at a time!

So, why another kettlebell book?

It would seem that everywhere you look there is a new book about kettlebells, so what's different about this one?

This book is a straightforward introduction to kettlebells for the beginner. It is written with the complete newbie in mind. It explains and illustrates the only exercises a newcomer needs to quickly and easily become proficient at kettlebell training, with no nonsense and no fuss.

I look forward to guiding you through this beginner's guide to kettlebell training, and hope that you find it easy to read, easy to understand, and easy to put into use.

THE HISTORY AND BACKGROUND OF KETTLEBELLS

The first known use of kettlebells was in Russia, near the start of the 1700's. They weren't called kettlebells back then, they were called girya. The kettlebell was most recently a military training tool used by the Soviet Red Army (who also invented Sambo – a deadly type of hand to hand combat).

Of course, 'old school' often comes back into fashion and a guy called Pavel Tsatsouline brought the kettlebell to the attention of American fitness enthusiasts. Pavel developed the first, and some would say only, real kettlebell certification. Many disagree with this certification's validity, in the same way that many people disagree with holding to the same training methods of karate masters from hundreds of years ago just because someone chose to pass down the information from generation to generation—all the time becoming like a game of Chinese Whispers.

Among those who have trained with Pavel or followed his instruction, there are a high number of followers who are almost religious in their fervor.

It wasn't long before marketers jumped on the bandwagon and a ton of celebrity endorsements and infomercials started taking control of the media. Unfortunately many of those promotions feel the need to distinguish themselves from others by creating new moves and giving them cutesy nicknames – diluting the real kettlebell training and removing a lot of the benefit. There are no such invented moves here. We will be training with the classic, old school methods that get results. You can safely leave the lycra pants where they belong ;-)

Kettlebell training is suited to both general fitness and many different sports-specific conditioning programs. Kettlebells are probably the most versatile pieces of training equipment you will ever find. With correct tuition it only takes a short time to gain expertise and feel the benefits. It is important to seek out instruction from a qualified teacher when using them for the first time. Poor exercise form can and sometimes does result in injury.

Before we move on I want to point out that although kettlebells are a simple tool, some of the exercises are deceptive. What seems like a very easy exercise can hide a complex set of movements that can't easily be shown in a book. For that reason I advise you to use this book as a supplement to a real world training class.

I don't believe anyone needs go to a class on an ongoing basis. Once you have attended a class and had an instructor view your form and correct it, I believe it's perfectly acceptable to continue your training with video/DVD/book training. If you enjoy the sociable element of a class or feel it is more beneficial to have that added level of accountability, then by all means a class is a good idea.

Please be careful about copying exercises from public sources such as YouTube. Many gyms have pulled kettlebells from their equipment due to people injuring themselves after copying incorrect form from YouTube videos. That's not to say there aren't valid training videos available on YouTube. There are – but you need to do your due diligence when selecting one.

BENEFITS OF KETTLEBELLS

Are kettlebells really the best – the "be all and end all of fat loss tools?"

The best exercise for fat loss is the one you do consistently—regardless of the tool. There is more than one way to the top of the mountain. That being said, kettlebells do offer more benefits than you might expect.

Kettlebells differ from conventional dumbbells by virtue of the fact that their weight is located some distance away from the handle, which is also thicker than that of most dumbbells. As a result, kettlebells are more difficult to move around and grip. The distance between where you grip and the centre of the kettlebell means the centre of gravity is not within your grip. While moving the kettlebell, the centre of gravity will constantly change and shift, which forces your muscles to adapt —and adapt quickly—to support each other in moving the bell. This support from other muscles is called compound exercise. Like money in the bank, compound is what gets greater results, faster.

This increased difficulty stimulates more muscle activity, which contributes to a higher rate of calorie burning than during other resistance exercise. Kettlebells lend themselves more readily than dumbbells or barbells to exercises involving swinging and ballistic movements, and therefore a greater number of muscle areas can be worked within the one exercise Compound exercises are a far greater stimulus to muscle than isolation exercise.

The swinging and ballistic movements involved in kettlebell training makes them an ideal tool for sports people, particularly martial artists, football players, runners—anyone who needs a combination of speed and power.

There are many exercises using kettlebells which are suitable for people with varying levels of experience and skill. This catalogue of kettlebell exercises provides a range of exercises for beginners.

Strength, flexibility and cardio all in one

Strength

It's obvious that lifting and moving a weight will build your strength, but what many girya love about the kettlebell is its (diversity). Training with a kettlebell builds strength, flexibility and cardio simultaneously. How's that for multi-tasking?

Flexibility

It may come as a surprise to you to think of kettlebells beyond a mere strength building tool, but they are effective in all round fitness. Kettlebell workout movements tend to include a lot of core movement and rotation. Due to the ballistic nature of these movements, kettlebells prove to be an effective core flexibility tool.

Cardio

Scientists at the University of Wisconsin were surprised to find that kettlebells are responsible for massive calorie burn. In research funded by the American Council of Exercise, research subjects burned an average of 272 calories – in only 20 minutes of exercise!
These amazing results aren't necessarily due to the size or shape of a kettlebell, but a combination of factors

which include the fact that kettlebell workouts are full body exercises and are typically done in an interval training format. You may have heard of this referred to as "high intensity interval training."

It's not as scary as it sounds. The idea behind high intensity interval training (HIIT) is that you train at as high a level of exertion as you can for a short period of time, rest for a shorter period of time, and repeat for a specified amount of time or repetitions. Getting the body used to the lack of recovery time between work times, forces it to respond more rapidly.

In the University of Wisconsin's research notes, Doctor Porcari states that the test results were equal to those achieved by running a 6 minute mile.

In addition, The ballistic nature of kettlebell lifting creates a challenge for the muscles that cardio workout alone does not do.

The weight of the kettlebell and the ballistic nature of the training combined with the extra effort required to steady the bell against an ever changing centre of gravity and the full body engagement in the exercises all combine to make kettlebell training a highly efficient form of calorie burning.

Why this constant fascination with keeping workouts short? If this is such a great workout why do people want to make it so short?

If you were a moviegoer in the '80s and '90s (or were lucky enough to own a VHS video player) you may recall many a montage made up of the hero spending hour after grueling hour doing hundreds of pushups, pull ups, bench presses, stretches, martial arts kata, and running for miles on end. Ehm, did they not have a job to go to? Seriously though, we have been conditioned to think that we need to spend hours at a time working out to get in great physical shape.

Consider this: do you think that people who work long shifts in police and enforcement—whose physical strength is almost a necessity—have the time to waste hours on keeping in shape? Absolutely not. High intensity interval training has become common place, and it has been shown that short bursts of high intensity training creates far better results than long, drawn out workouts, which do little more than fatigue the body.

Look at most dogs. They are generally lean and muscular and capable of rapid explosive movement (unless their owners are obese, in which case the poor dog stands a good chance of being fat too). But aside from doing downward dog stretches and short bursts of running, what does a dog do for the day? Eats from time to time and sleeps all day!

We may be dressed up in suits and have a medulla oblongata at the top of our brain stems, but we are largely still nothing more than animals and physically it would be well to remember that. Short, intense periods of exercise followed by the necessary amount of recuperation get us to our fitness goals much faster than wasting a lot of time wearing ourselves out.

Get warmed up, get moving, get your body good and hot and your heart pumping and keep it that way for 20 minutes and you have done a great workout. The key is in making sure to be consistent. All those 20 minute workouts add up to a much better result than a two hour "power" workout done less often.

A Note of Caution

Because kettlebell exercises differ considerably from other resistance and weight-bearing exercises for reasons outlined above, care should be taken by those beginning a program involving them.

Anyone with back and shoulder problems, or a weak core, should consult a physician or appropriately qualified medical practitioner before commencing an exercise program involving kettlebells as some exercises if done incorrectly, can have a negative effect on any pre-existing problem areas.

A qualified personal trainer or fitness class instructor who has experience with (and, ideally, certification with) kettlebells should select, demonstrate and monitor appropriate exercises for the beginner.

Those who are accustomed to training with heavier weights, such as used in muscle building programs, should bear in mind that the vast majority of kettlebell exercises are compound rather than isolating in nature, and often involve explosive movement.

The correct weight for your kettlebell or how many kettlebells you require will depend on your fitness goal.

A lighter weight of kettlebell should be selected to begin with, and heavier kettlebells should not be used until perfect form is achieved with the lighter ones. This is an important point.

In his book, Enter The Kettlebell! Strength Secret of The Soviet Supermen, Pavel Tsatsouline recommends that when learning a new routine, girya should practice the movements for the exercise separately from the actual workout.

The idea is that you shouldn't overwhelm yourself with trying to work out and learn the exercises at the same time. And it's a valid point.

Safety Tip!

Make sure you work out somewhere you can't easily damage your floors, or else you are using a good solid mat. If you feel the kettlebell slipping from your hand, get your feet out of the way! Forget about the floor, keep your feet free from injury.

SUGGESTED KETTLEBELL WEIGHTS

Everyone is different, and while some guys might find a 12kg bell challenging enough to start with, others will find heavier kettlebells immediately fit their ability.

Here is the suggested starting weight for anyone beginning a kettlebell routine. Included are suggestions for what weights you should consider using as a set when you begin to graduate to heavier weights. This isn't an immediate concern. For now, pick the weight that seems good to you and one you can comfortably hold overhead.

Current Strength	Starting Weight	Suggested Set of Kettlebells
Average Female	18lb / 8kg	12lb, 26lb, 35lb / 8kg, 12kg, 16kg
Strong Female	26lb / 12kg	26lb, 35lb, 44lb / 12kg, 16kg, 20kg
Average Male	35lb / 16kg	35lb, 44lb, 53lb / 16kg, 20kg, 24kg
Strong Male	44lb / 20kg	44lb, 53lb, 70lb / 20kg, 24kg, 32kg
Very Strong Male	53lb / 24kg	53lb, 70lb, 88lb / 24kg, 32kg, 40kg

As you can see, kettlebells come with big differences in weight between one size and the next, which is very different to how standard barbell and dumbbell exercises work. While you may be more familiar, in theory at least, with resistance training methods that gradually increase the weight by a pound or two as strength increases, each kettlebell is 4kg heavier than the last. The standard beginners is called a "pood" which is the Russian measure of approx. 16kg. Because of the difference in weight from one kettlebell to another, going too heavy too soon is a bad idea. Too light is a bad idea, and we will get to that shortly.

Most people's first concern is what will happen when they are comfortable with their starting weight? Will they be forced into spending more money and allocating more floor space to bigger and bigger kettlebells? If this is a concern for you, don't worry. There are a range of techniques involved with kettlebell training that allow for a very varied array of challenges. When doing pushups for example, it's possible to increase the resistance against your body by elevating the feet, clapping at the apex of the movement and so on. Similarly, with kettlebells, we can use one weight in many ways to create extra difficulty. The need to constantly stabilize the centre of gravity works incredibly well in creating a myriad of different challenges.

Note: I feel compelled to mention that women in particular, make a common mistake regarding the starting weight of their kettlebells. Unfortunately, many of the "celebrity" DVDs that have flooded the supermarket shelves come with advice that women should start with a 6kg bell. Many even bundle a nice little pink 6kg bell in with their product.

This is dangerous!

Please understand something about the ballistic nature of kettlebell training: unlike traditional western weight training where we are told not to swing the weight, we are encouraged to do so in many (not all) kettlebell routines. With traditional dumbbells and barbells, swinging the weight can lead to injury because the centre of gravity is within the weights themselves. If you were to swing one and lost control, the COG (centre of gravity) would pull your limb further from its range of motion than it should and place you at risk of injury.

With a kettlebell, we can swing the bell. To tell the truth, with many kettlebell exercises we don't even need to have perfect form to get a lot of benefit from them, because the weight of the kettlebell combined with the external COG automatically places limits on how far we can extend our movement. Our brain often has problems with evaluating the weight of an object compared to its size.

What seems like something we should be able to move as far as we want isn't the case when it's an iron ball.

If we use the correct weight and get carried away in our workout, it's not possible to over extend our muscles, because the weight of the kettlebell will prevent us from doing so. But if we are working out with a kettlebell that is too light, we can easily hyperextend (overextend) a limb and risk injury to the muscle.

Don't be afraid of a kettlebell. Don't think that by deliberately choosing a lighter kettlebell you will get "more of a cardio effect" from your training. This is a fallacy. You will get a cardio workout regardless. Another point with tiny kettlebells is - if it's not moving around its COG and forcing your supporting muscles to engage, what's the point of using it? You may as well just pick up a small dumbbell and forget all about kettlebells.

OTHER EQUIPMENT

One of the reasons kettlebells are spoken of so highly is the lack of need for any further equipment. I choose to disagree with that and will explain what other equipment I recommend and why:

A floor mat. If you are training at home you will need this for future exercises (not covered in this beginner's guide) that will require you to lay on your back, or get on your knees. Not only will these save wear and tear on your body, but it will prevent you destroying your workout floor with sweat when it starts coming off you in buckets!

Weight lifting shoes. The nature of kettlebell training is one of finely balanced reaction within your body to the external stimulus – I can't stress enough how the movement of the centre of gravity causes supporting muscles to work.

All the supporting muscles root themselves in the core. It is for this reason that the standard training footwear, with its gel insoles are a bad idea. They prevent the kettlebell user from correctly using their core and the imbalances this cause will only have a negative effect on their training.

At home I recommend you train in your bare feet (note: stockinged feet and sweaty workout mats are a bad mix).

If however, you want to rain at a gym, weight lifting shoes are perfect. They are flat with no gel. Also see martial arts shoes which are similar and for similar reasons.

A foam pad. I got mine from a gardening centre as it was intended for gardeners to kneel on for comfort. Thing is, I own a set of kettlebells – 2 x 12kg, one 16kg and a 20kg – which don't work well with wooden flooring at home. Save your floor, buy a foam knee gardening thingy.

Weight lifting gloves. As you progress you will find that the kettlebell can cause calluses on your hands if you are not using perfect form. This can be corrected by wearing weight lifting gloves to protect your hands.

A timer. A stopwatch will be awkward with this kind of workout, but it is important that you are able to time yourself correctly. No need to spend money on this if you already own a laptop, iPad or smart phone (which, if you're reading the kindle version of this, is a given).

Have you been put off by the ridiculous cost of workout timers? Me too. That's why I tried and tested many, many types of free timers until I arrived back at Gymboss and found out that although the Gymboss can be bought as a standalone timer, it is also available as a free app in the Google Play store. It has all the functionality of the one you would otherwise spend your dollars on, and is highly customizable. There you go, that's money saved straight away!

A skipping rope. This isn't necessary at all, but sometimes I use skipping to warm up for my workout. It only needs a few minutes, costs very little and takes up virtually no space - and like kettlebells there is enormous benefit from a very small investment of time. A perfect combination.

STRETCHING AND WARM-UP

Kettlebell exercises can place great demands on joint flexibility and strength as well as coordination. Therefore warm-ups for kettlebell routines should include specific stretches and engagement of all joints: wrists, elbows, shoulders, hips, knees and ankles.

These stretches should be made up of a combination of static stretches (holding the stretch for up to two minutes per stretch), 'ballistic' stretches (a number of repetitions moving in and out of end ranges, e,g. kicks and punches) and coordination exercises which integrate lower and upper body movements (e.g. jumping jacks).

Always warm up before stretching. Stretching your muscles without a warm up can result in injury. Jumping Jacks are perfect if you don't want to skip. Pushups and lunges are also perfectly good as warm ups.

Move from a warm up to ballistic stretches and then to static stretching. Static stretching can place a lot of pressure on your muscles if they are cold. Remember, the whole point of stretching isn't just "to be flexible" – it's a safety guard against injury. Injury that can very easily be caused inadvertently by overextending a limb, or moving a muscle too far or too fast, causing it to tear.

Workout smarter, and harder (I adapted that from my old corporate job, but I don't think they would appreciate how it reads now).

When exercising with kettlebells, a clear working space of around 3m or 9 ft is ideal. Keep away from glass, ornaments, or anything your wife or husband values more than you!

BEGINNER'S KETTLEBELL WORKOUT PROGRAM

The beginner workout program consists of a circuit, and is based on time. This will allow you become familiar with the exercises without the pressure of having to perform a specified number of exercises. Simply do the exercise and do it correctly for as many times as you can while keeping good form. As you progress, you will naturally fill the time with more repetitions.

Beginner Level Workout

Order of Exercises:

The exercises in each circuit are listed in the order in which they should be performed. The exercises are described and illustrated in the pages that follow the workout description.

Number of Circuits per Workout and Rests

I recommend repeating the circuit three times, depending on your fitness level. After completing one exercise, go straight into the next one. Short rests of between 60 and 90 seconds can be taken in between circuits.

Repetitions and Time Taken

This workout is entirely time-based, meaning you

perform as many repetitions as possible within the nominated time limit.

The Workout

Objective: To increase muscular strength and endurance in as wide a variety of muscle group areas as possible while also improving cardiovascular performance

Total time taken (estimated, excluding rest time): less than 20mins, subject to length of time per exercise. Do each exercise for 30 seconds then rest for 30 seconds before attempting the next exercise.

Number of circuits to be performed in one workout: 3-5. Start at 3 and build to 5 over time. Similarly, you may decrease the rest time as your ability increases. Your ultimate goal is to hit 45 seconds of work and 15 seconds of rest for each exercise.

Exercise	Amount of Time	Important notes
Two-handed Kettlebell Swing	30-45sec	Remember to drive hips forward explosively (but smoothly) while swinging the kettlebell forward
Deadlift	30-45sec	Pull kettlebells towards your stomach maintaining spine-neutral position (back straight, chest out) and keeping your elbows tucked in
Alternating Kettlebell Press	30-45sec	A good alternative to bench presses but demands a compound wrist and arm movement.
Woodman's Chop	30-45sec	Remember to keep your lower back in its natural arch and to pivot.
Goblet squat/Front Squat	30-45sec	Squat as low as you can and drive back up through your heels.

Two Handed Kettlebell Swing

Skill Level: Beginner

Main Muscle Groups Worked:

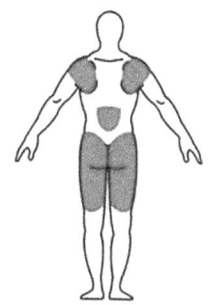
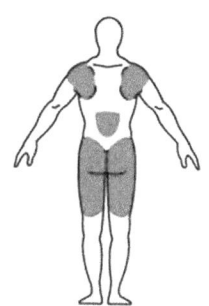

Lower Back	Biceps	Adductors
Middle Back	Triceps	Quadriceps
Trapezius	Forearms	Calves
Latissimus Dorsi	Abdominals	Shoulders
Gluteus Maximus	Obliques	Hips
	Chest	Hamstrings

David Lynch

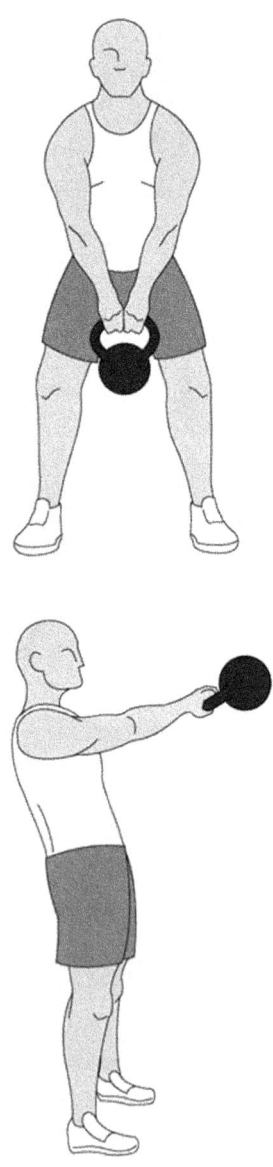

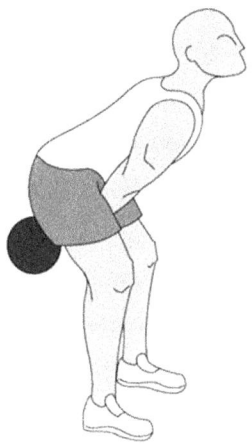

Exercise Steps

Stand in spine-neutral position with feet slightly wider than shoulder-width apart.

Hold kettlebell with both hands, palms down, arms in front of body.

Bend knees slightly and thrust hips back, as for a squat, but don't go down as far.

Maintaining a fluid motion, drive hips forward explosively while swinging the kettlebell forwards and to shoulder height, engaging hips and glutes all the time. The hips and glutes, rather than the arms, should be driving the kettlebell forward.

Lower kettlebell back down between legs and repeat swinging motion for 12-15 repetitions, or according to your particular program and weight of kettlebell.

KB Swing Expert Tip #1

When swinging a kettlebell with one arm is very important to prevent injury by co-coordinating your other arm. It's not difficult to do and it will ensure solid and safe training. When you swing the kettlebell forward with one arm, move your other arm forward as if it is holding a phantom kettlebell. Similarly when swinging your arm back between your leg, continue the movement of your weight-free arm so that the movement finishes behind your back, parallel to the arm holding the kettlebell.

Keeping both arms moving together like this will prevent any injury that might otherwise be caused by twisting in opposing directions.

KB Swing Expert Tip #2

It's important during a swing that you keep your back straight and don't crouch or bend too much. There is a slight difference between a kettlebell swing and a standard squat. The easiest way I find of ensuring correct form is to keep your leg from the foot to your knee in a vertical line throughout the exercise. This will ensure that the rest of the body movement is automatically correct.

Kettlebell Deadlift

Skill Level: Beginner

Main Muscle Groups Worked:

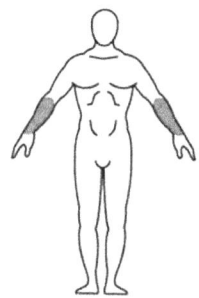 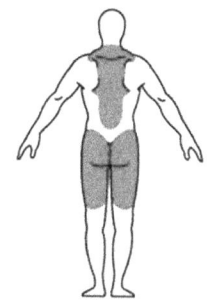

Lower Back
Middle Back
Trapezius
Latissimus Dorsi
Shoulders
Gluteus Maximus

Biceps
Triceps
Forearms
Abdominals
Obliques
Chest

Adductors
Quadriceps
Calves
Hips
Hamstrings

David Lynch

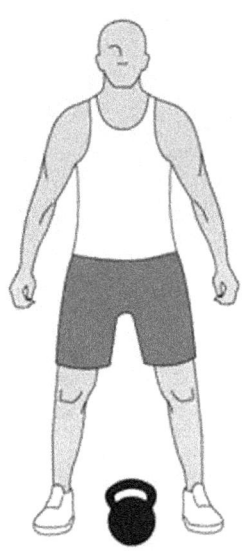

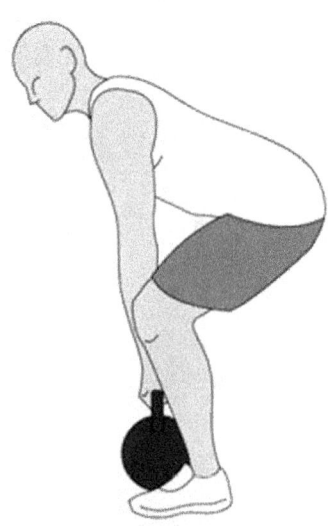

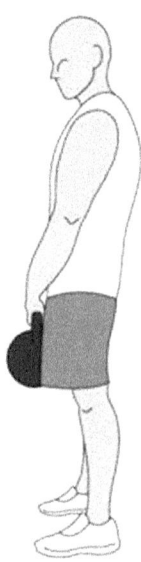

Exercise Steps

Stand with the kettlebell between your feet.

Bend your knees to squat down and take the kettlebell with both hands. Maintain spine neutral position (back remains flat).

Engage your core, tighten your glutes, and keep your arms extended as you raise your body by pushing up through your feet. Don't pull the kettlebell up with your arms – just let it come along with you, until you come to a standing position.

Lower the kettlebell back down to the ground again by

bending your knees and keeping your arms extended. Aim for 12-15 repetitions, maintaining proper form throughout.

Goblet Squat/Front Squat

Skill Level: Beginner

Main Muscle Groups Worked:

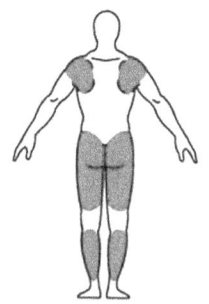 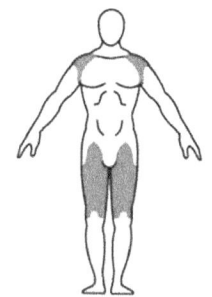

Lower Back
Middle Back
Trapezius
Latissimus Dorsi
Shoulders

Biceps
Triceps
Forearms
Abdominals
Obliques
Chest

Adductors
Quadriceps
Calves
Gluteus Maximus
Hips
Hamstrings

David Lynch

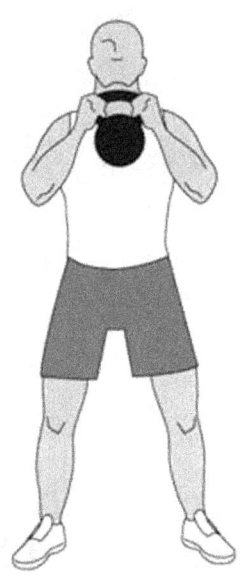

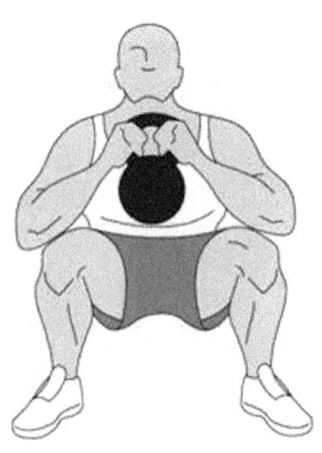

Exercise Steps

Hold a kettlebell by the handle close to your chest and assume a comfortable stance.

Bring your knees out as you squat down to bring the kettlebell between them.

Looking straight ahead at all times, squat as low as you can.

Pause at the bottom of the squat.

Keep your head and chest up, with your back in spine-neutral position (straight).

Rise back up by driving through your heels.

Repeat for 12-15 repetitions.

Kettlebell Woodman's Chop

Skill Level: Beginner

Main Muscle Groups Worked:

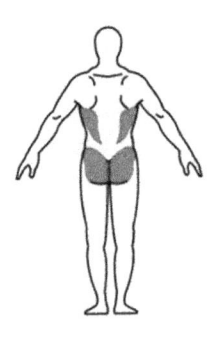

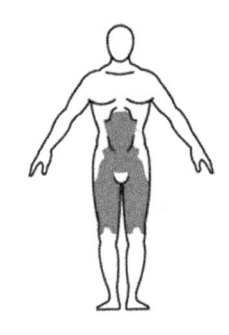

Lower Back	Biceps	Adductors
Middle Back	Triceps	Quadriceps
Trapezius	Forearms	Calves
Latissimus Dorsi	Abdominals	Gluteus Maximus
Shoulders	Obliques	Hips
	Chest	Hamstrings

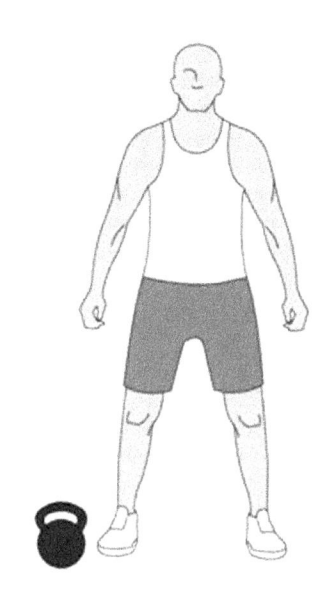

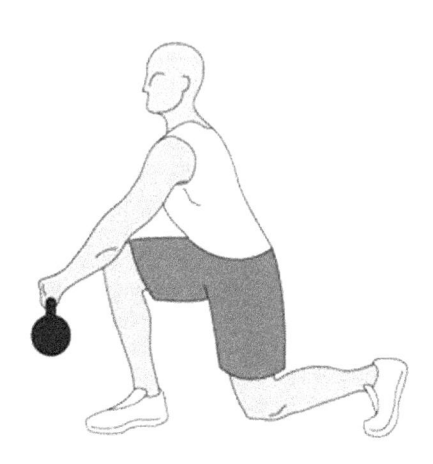

Kettlebell Workouts for Beginners

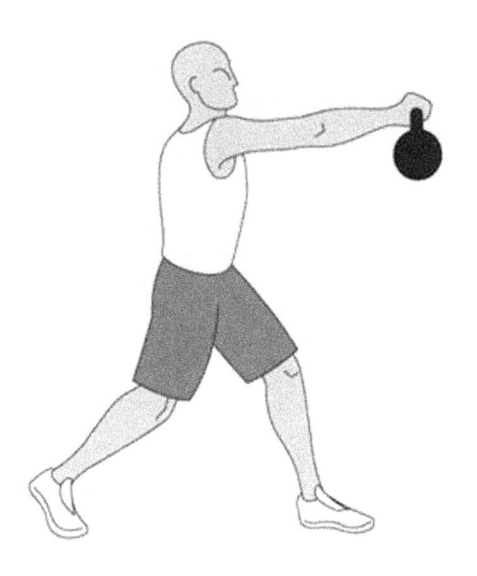

Exercise Steps

Stand with your feet outside shoulder width with a kettlebell on the floor to your right side.

Keeping your lower back in its natural arch, pivot your feet to the right and bend down and pick up the kettlebell by the handle

Raise it as you pivot and twist to the left, stopping when the bell is at chest height.

Return the weight to the floor. Repeat 12-15 repetitions per side.

Once you have become familiar with the beginner program it's natural you will want to progress, and so I am including a Beginner-Intermediate exercise, and Intermediate and an Advanced exercise, so that you can progress without having to necessarily buy another book.

David Lynch

One Handed Kettlebell Swing

Skill Level: Beginner-Intermediate

Main Muscle Groups Worked:

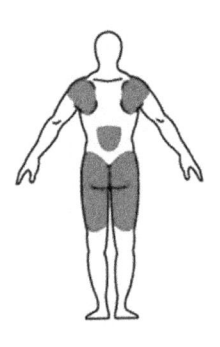

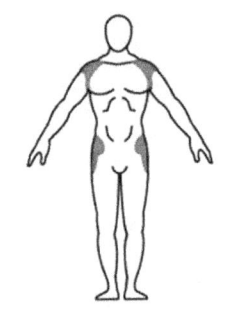

Lower Back	Biceps	Adductors
Middle Back	Triceps	Quadriceps
Trapezius	Forearms	Calves
Latissimus Dorsi	Abdominals	Gluteus Maximus
Shoulders	Obliques	Hips
	Chest	Hamstrings

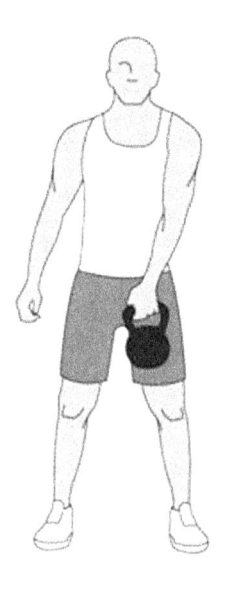

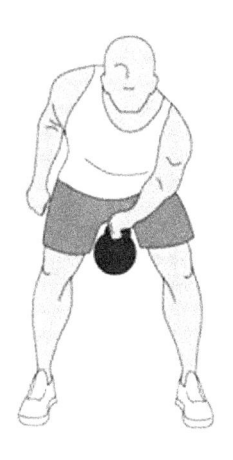

Kettlebell Workouts for Beginners

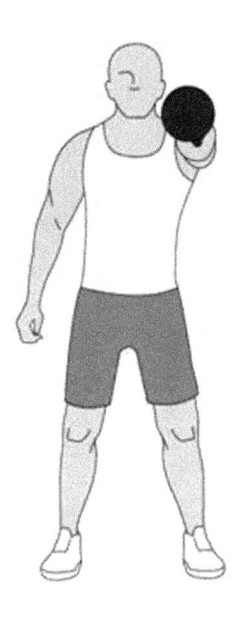

Exercise Steps

Stand in spine-neutral position with feet slightly more than shoulder-width apart.

Hold kettlebell with one hand, palm down and arms in front of body.

Bend knees slightly and thrust hips back, as for a squat, but don't go down as far.

Maintaining a fluid motion, drive hips forward explosively while swinging the kettlebell forwards with one hand to shoulder height, engaging hips and glutes all the time.

Swing the other arm out at the same time to maintain your balance and help drive momentum. The hips and glutes, rather than your arm, should be driving the kettlebell forward.

When the kettlebell reaches its highest point it should hang "dead" in the air for a moment before it starts its downward movement. At this point take it in your other hand and allow it to swing down between your legs.

Swing it out again, focusing on the hip thrust to power it out.

Repeat swinging motion for 12-15 repetitions per side, or according to your particular program and weight of kettlebell.

Kettlebell Rotating Lunge

Skill Level: Intermediate

Main Muscle Groups Worked:

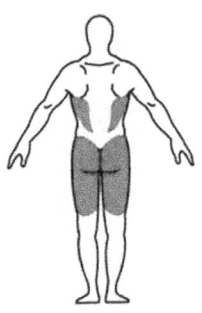

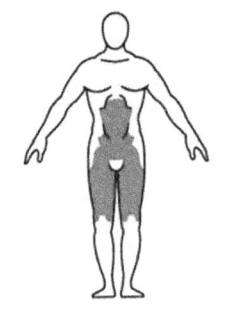

Lower Back	Biceps	Adductors
Middle Back	Triceps	Quadriceps
Trapezius	Forearms	Calves
Latissimus Dorsi	Abdominals	Gluteus Maximus
Shoulders	Obliques	Hips
	Chest	Hamstrings

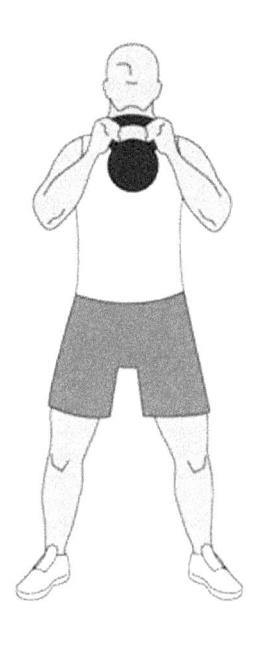

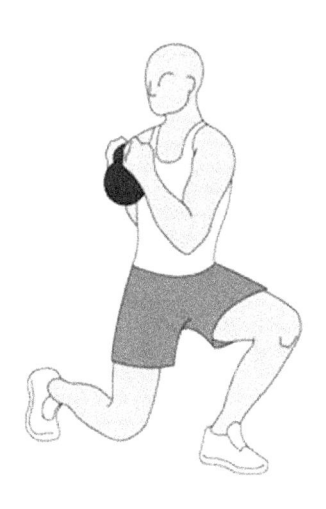

Kettlebell Workouts for Beginners

Exercise Steps

Stand with your feet shoulder-width apart holding a kettlebell with both hands in front of your chest.

Step forward with your left leg and lower into a lunge, simultaneously rotating your upper body toward the right wall.

Drive through the left heel and return to the starting position.

Repeat for 12-15 repetitions on each side.

As you become accustomed to the movement, you can increase the difficulty by turning your torso the opposite direction.

Kettlebell Push-Up with Row

Skill Level: Advanced

Main Muscle Groups Worked:

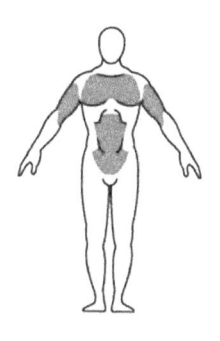

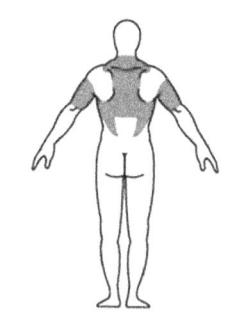

Lower Back	Biceps	Adductors
Middle Back	Triceps	Quadriceps
Trapezius	Forearms	Calves
Latissimus Dorsi	Abdominals	Gluteus Maximus
Shoulders	Obliques	Hips
	Chest	Hamstrings

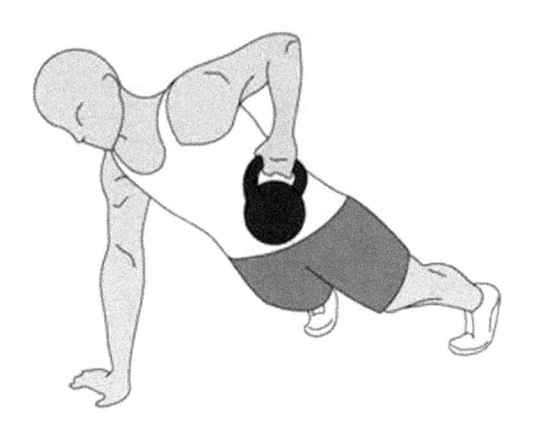

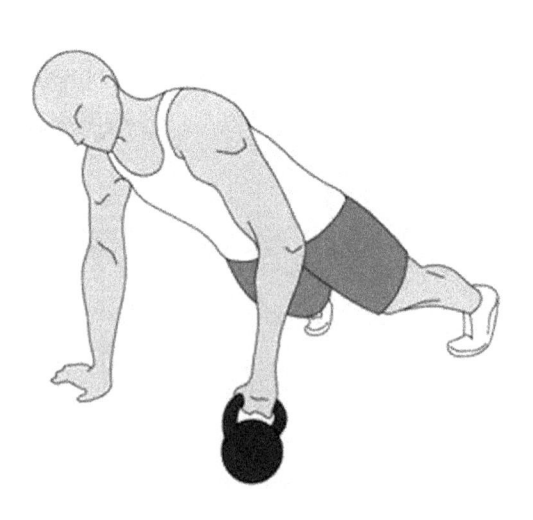

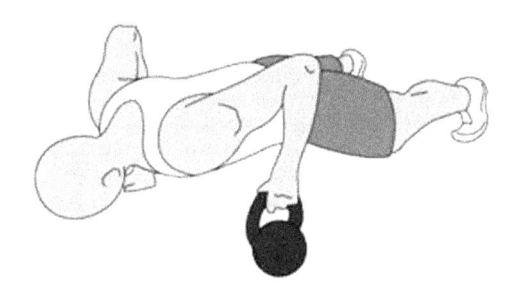

Exercise Steps

Begin in a push-up position with the left arm holding a kettlebell.

Perform a push-up and hold at the top.

Squeeze your shoulder blades together to lift your left elbow about 15 cm above your body as you pull the kettlebell up to your chest.

TAKING YOUR TRAINING FURTHER

Combining kettlebells with bodyweight training can help move your training forward and is often a great way to get over any training plateaus. Kettlebell and bodyweight exercise complement each other very nicely. Neither needs a great deal of complexity, which means any number of quick and easy to understand workout varieties are possible.

There are no rules for combining the two workouts. Here's one I suggest:

Begin with the kettlebell swing, performing 3 sets of 25 swings with a short rest in between each set.

Continue with 20 pushups.

Perform a goblet squat for 3 sets of 30 seconds.

Do a further 20 pushups.

Continue in this manner with your own choice of further kettlebell exercises until you have completed four sets of pushups.

Adding A Second Kettlebell

Many people like to add a second kettlebell to explore other exercises before moving on to intermediate and advanced workouts. Here are two additional exercises if you choose to do this.

Two-Arm Kettlebell Row

Skill Level: Beginner-Intermediate

Main Muscle Groups Worked:

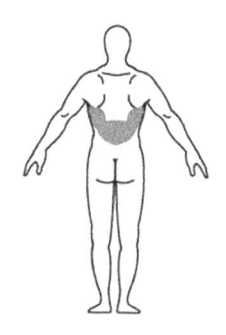

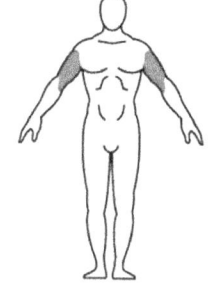

Lower Back	Biceps	Adductors
Middle Back	Triceps	Quadriceps
Trapezius	Forearms	Calves
Latissimus Dorsi	Abdominals	Gluteus Maximus
Shoulders	Obliques	Hips
	Chest	Hamstrings

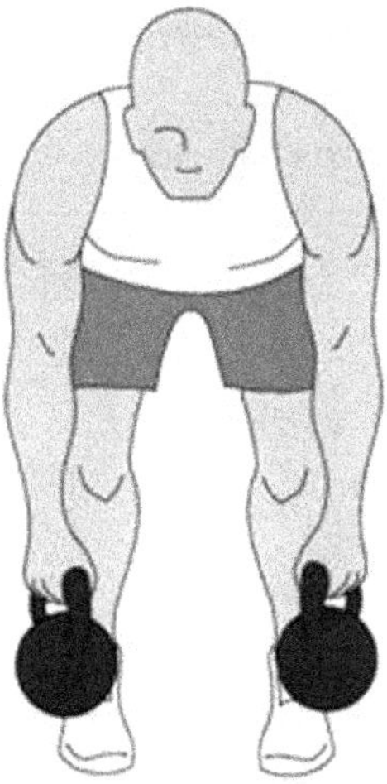

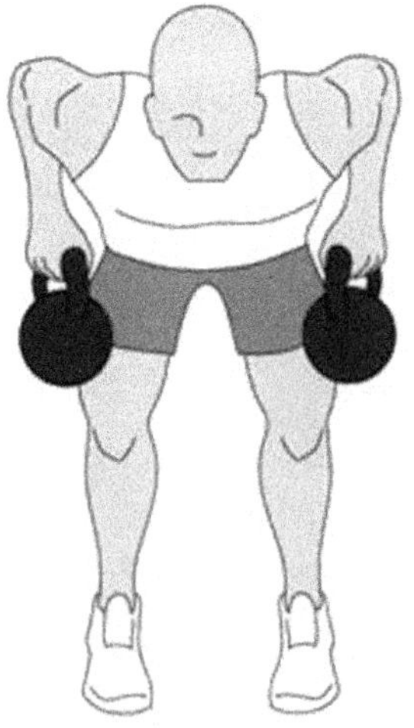

Exercise Steps

Take two kettlebells and place them in front of your feet.

Bend knees slightly.

Bend over to pick up the kettlebells while maintaining spine neutral position.

Pull kettlebells towards your stomach maintaining spine-neutral position (back straight, chest out) and keeping your elbows tucked in.

Lower kettlebells and repeat for 8-10 repetitions.

Alternating Kettlebell Press

Skill Level: Intermediate

Main Muscle Groups Worked:

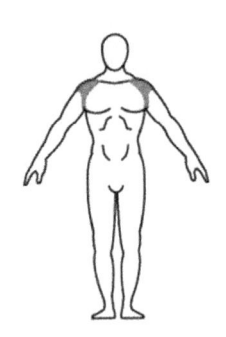

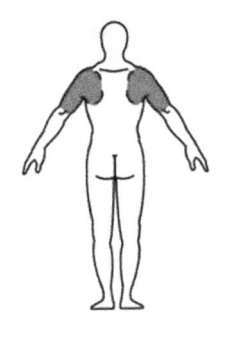

Lower Back	Biceps	Adductors
Middle Back	Triceps	Quadriceps
Trapezius	Forearms	Calves
Latissimus Dorsi	Abdominals	Gluteus Maximus
Shoulders	Obliques	Hips
	Chest	Hamstrings

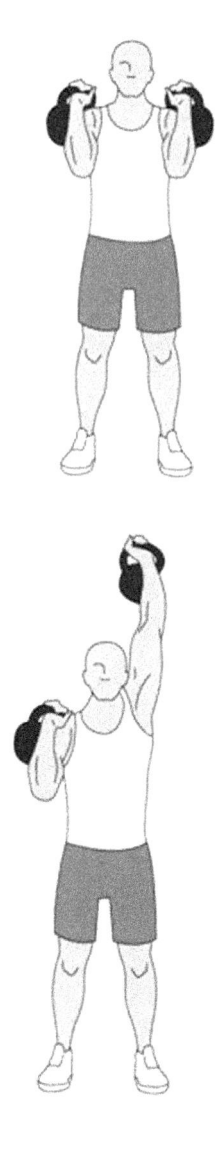

Kettlebell Workouts for Beginners

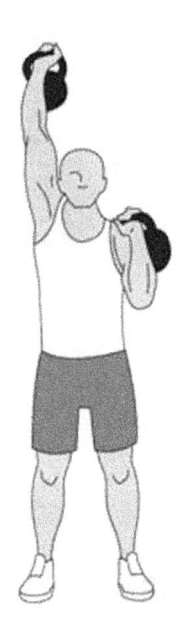

Exercise Steps

Bring two kettlebells to your shoulders using the clean motion.

Press one kettlebell directly overhead by extending your arm through your elbow, turning your wrist so that your palms face forward. Hold the other kettlebell stationary on your shoulder.

Lower the pressed kettlebell back down to your shoulder and immediately press the other kettlebell up with your arm.

Repeat alternating presses for 8-10 repetitions per side.

NUTRITION

I hate giving nutritional advice. There are so many different theories about what works and what doesn't and why or why not they don't, that I get incredibly bored with the arguments that follow.

There are however some universal points I'd like you to consider if you want to get the most from your training. To effectively build muscle and lose fat, you absolutely must pay attention to your diet. There is no ambiguity in this statement.

Universal Truth #1: The old way of looking at diet as the food pyramid many of us were taught by the school or government system is wrong. Forget all about that stuff about having a large base of carbohydrates and moving up to a point where you eat a small amount of protein.

That system was brought about as a marketing plan. At one point in the United States there was a surplus of vegetables. The idea came about that everyone should get their "five a day" or else suffer the negative health consequences. Phooey! Also, people were historically not so well off financially as they are today (though the ever increasing divide between the well off and those less fortunate is a topic of debate for another day). So the more expensive food – meat – was suggested to be eaten in small amounts.

Traditionally the idea has been that lots of carbs gives lots of energy and then we have protein in small amounts and we should avoid fat at all costs or else we would become obese.

Not so! We are generally better off eating good fats and protein. These help keep our tissue flexible, our brains active and our nerves in good shape. I understand there are vegetarians out there, but protein does not have to be meat. Did you know that rice and peas together make a complete protein -and they are cheap too!

To summarize: ***Ditch the carbs, eat fats and protein.***

Universal Truth #2: Aside from ensuring to eat plenty of fats and protein, how your diet affects you is extremely individual in nature. There are people for whom one type of food is a fountain of youth and energy, while for others it is poison that saps their energy and expands their waistline. We are all different. Don't just blindly follow a method of nutrition based on what someone else tells you is correct. You may even break Universal Nutrition Rule #1 if you disagree with me. Go ahead – I give you full permission.

To achieve a good diet you need to try different things. While the Paleo diet appeals to me a lot, the only diet I have ever tried that has had a positive mental and physical effect on me has been the 2 Day Diet (available in paperback and on Kindle).

I suggest at least trying it for a month to see if it works for you. Personally, I lost 5kg in the first two weeks and then applied that principles to a one day diet once I got where I wanted to be. This also included Faturday – which for me coincides with Saturday – the day I get to eat and drink any amount of anything I want. Guinness Extra Stout make a lot of money from me on Faturdays!

Some of the benefits I found with this method of dieting were:

I didn't need to tax my brain with minute calculations of calorie intake

If I really craved something like a chocolate bar I just thought, I'll have it on Faturday. Often, by the time Faturday came round I had forgotten all about that temporary whim

I became more aware of why I was eating. On the two diet days I realized that often I wasn't really hungry. In reality I was going to the fridge out of boredom or to fulfill some emotional need for comfort. There are better ways of fulfilling emotional needs.

Universal Nutrition Rule #3: Weight loss, building muscle and/or toning up is much more to do with diet than it is exercise. I would hesitate to put exact numbers on it, but in my opinion I would say that how fat or fit we are is 80% diet and 20% exercise. Another reason to put 20 minutes into getting fit compared to wasting hours just tiring yourself out.

Don't become disheartened and think there's little point to exercise if it is only a quarter as important as exercise is. Firstly, that's just my estimation, and secondly, if you haven't heard about the 80/20 rule, it's a rule of thumb that an Italian by the name of Pareto came up with and it is widely used in business today - basically 80% of your results will come from 20% of your activity. The 80% that is your diet is stoking the fire that the 20% of exercise uses to burn away the fat and build muscle. You definitely need to combine both diet and exercise for results.

How Eating Fat Will Help You Get Fit

Dietary fats are something many people wrongly believe they should avoid when trying to lead a healthy lifestyle. However, the truth is that with the exception of trans fats, dietary fats are essential for good health and something that you should be eating regularly. Let's take a detailed look at the four main types of dietary fats and provide you with a full overview of each one.

Saturated Fats

Saturated fats are probably the most feared of the four fats with many sources claiming that they lead to clogged arteries, heart disease and more. However, the truth is that saturated fats are essential for good health and without them your body would not function properly. The roles of saturated fats in the body include:

Protecting against heart disease

Strengthening your bones

Strengthening your cell wells

Strengthening your immune system

Strengthening your nervous system

Strengthening your vital organs

Animal products such as butter, dairy and red meat are excellent sources of saturated fats. However, if you're a vegetarian, avocado, coconut and other types of nuts are a great way to fill up on this nutrient.

Monounsaturated Fats

Monounsaturated fats keep your blood healthy and

also protect your body against a number of unpleasant ailments. The list below highlights the main functions of monounsaturated fats in your body:

Improving blood glucose regulation

Increasing blood levels of HDL cholesterol (which helps to clear LDL cholesterol from your artery walls)

Increasing the rate at which your body burns fat

Protecting against cancer

Protecting against inflammation

Reducing blood levels of LDL cholesterol (which builds up in your artery walls and restricts blood flow)

Monounsaturated fats are almost exclusively found in pant based foods with avocados, olive oil, most nuts and most seeds containing high levels of these health boosting fats.

Polyunsaturated Fats

Polyunsaturated fats can be broken down into two main types – omega 3 essential fatty acids (EFAs) and omega 6 EFAs. They benefit your body in the following ways:

Boosting your brain

Boosting your skin

Boosting your vision

Protecting against cancer

Protecting against heart disease

Strengthening your bones

Some of the best food sources of omega 3 EFAs include cold water fish (such as anchovies and salmon), dairy products and flaxseed oil. Some of the best food sources of omega 6 EFAs include most types of nuts and sunflower seed oil.

Trans Fats

Unlike the three dietary fats listed above, trans fats are not required by your body and consuming them can actually be damaging to your health. They are a man-made, artificial type of fat which food manufacturers use to extend the shelf life of their products and something you want to avoid where possible. The negative symptoms of consuming trans fats include:

Increased Alzheimer's risk

Increased cancer risk

CONCLUSION

Congratulations, not only on picking up this book to help create a better, fitter, happier you – but on finishing the book.

I am glad to have been of help, and I wish you every success in your fitness goals. If you enjoyed this book and found it helpful, I would really appreciate it if you could leave a review for me and point out what you found helpful. I will be following up with a book for intermediate training and any feedback you leave in your review will help me understand what people find useful.

All the best,
David

ABOUT THE AUTHOR

David Lynch began his fitness journey at the age of 16 when he started copying his parents during their marathon training runs. A misguided attempt at muscle building with an old fashioned bullworker and chest expander followed after watching Rocky. As the years went by his knowledge of fitness increased. Unfortunately his fashion sense took longer to develop and he pleads guilty to having worn gym gear that would cause even the cast of Flashdance to cringe. David ran his first marathon at the age of 30 so as to be able to say he did it. He followed up with a further 7 marathons. His kettlebell training began in 2012 and he plans to continue writing more helpful books on the topic.

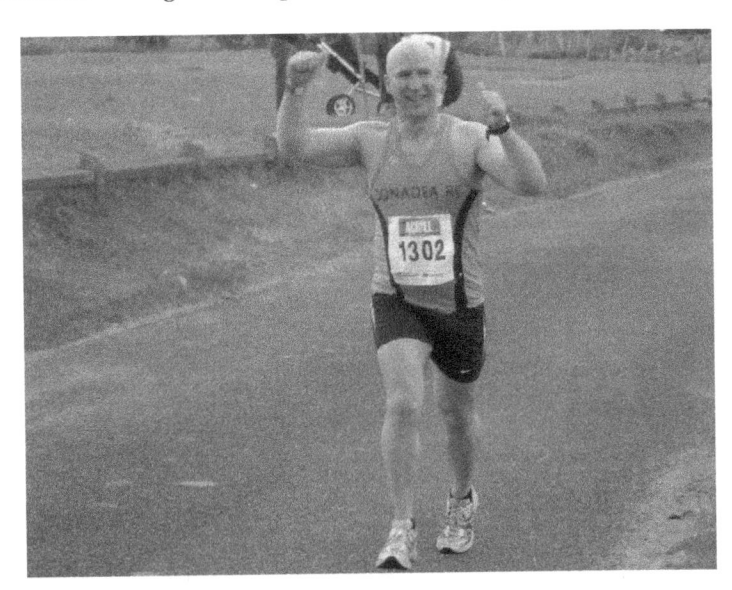